I0440544

Your Mid-Afternoon Energy Crash and What You Can Do About It

TOFFLER NIEMUTH

DEDICATION

To the countless people that will resonate with the story
shared herein, this book is for you.

CONTENTS

ACKNOWLEDGMENTS

Many thanks to all the volunteer editors who offered their input and feedback on this book: my grandparents, Dean and Betty Jean, my mom, Marcia, Jane Newby, Anna Gruter, Luke Chao, Harper Piver, Michael Hwan, and Alexander Rinehart.

INTRODUCTION

Heavy eyelids, foggy brain, slumped in your chair, staring mindlessly, and you just read the same sentence for the 4th time…

That's the mid-afternoon slump. Coffee crash. 3 o'clock lull.

Whatever you call it, most people have experienced it at some point: that dip in energy and focus, sometimes accompanied by sleepiness, irritability, or boredom, that usually occurs between 1-5 pm.

I, too, have suffered from the mid-afternoon slump. I'd be at work all morning, eat lunch, and then middle of the afternoon, about 3 pm, my energy would sink. I'd have a difficult time concentrating and even seeing straight. I'd be desperate for a nap or something else to restore my energy.

Does this sound familiar?

Undoubtedly it does. I've talked to hundreds of people who resonate with this story and who are just like you, looking for explanations, but more importantly, solutions.

This book is the result of many years of learning about and trying to understand the complex factors that result in low energy mid-afternoon.

Initially I sought a 'grab-n-go' solution, a fix-it-and-be-done option. But much to my dismay and disappointment, there wasn't any. I continued exploring the causes, trying to understand the lifestyle factors at play, and testing various scenarios to prevent, or at least, relieve the mid-afternoon slump.

Through the exploratory and learning journey, I was still searching for a solution that provided the satisfaction of immediate gratification I originally hoped for. In a later section, I'll explain what I finally developed that works for me. But more importantly, I want you to have an understanding of the surrounding issues so you can feel great all through the afternoon on your own accord.

In this book, I've summed up for the most common reasons for the afternoon slump, and the most sure-fire, safe, and healthy ways (discovered after much trial and error), to get through that lull and to prevent it.

Part I

WHY YOUR ENERGY CRASHES MID-AFTERNOON

COFFEE

Yes, coffee, the holy grail of alertness, concentration, and waking up in the morning may actually be the prime cause of your mid-afternoon suffering. Coffee gets you up and going in the morning because of caffeine. But what happens when the caffeine effect wears off or you build up a tolerance to it?

Most people drink coffee throughout the morning, drinking less and less by lunchtime. Though the caffeine effect can can hit within 45 minutes, its effect typically lasts 2.5 to 4.5 hours.[1]

That means, if you had your last cup at 10 am, by 1 or 2 pm, you're struggling to stay awake and alert, much the same way you were when you woke up. You feel like you've hit a wall when the caffeine effect has worn off.

Coffee can also have negative impacts on sleep quality, which further perpetuates the need for a morning jolt.

CARBOHYDRATES

You eat some carbohydrates--a bowl of pasta, sandwich with multigrain bread, a cookie, or two, or three--and you get a nice spike in blood sugar (because all carbohydrates, except fiber, are converted directly to sugar). Then your body releases insulin to deal with all that sugar, storing it in muscles, fat, and the liver. Once insulin has effectively dealt with the sugar in your blood, again your eyelids feel heavy, brain is foggy, and your energy is lower than before you ate (since blood sugar has come back down).

Low blood sugar means you feel tired, slow, and often irritable. This feeling is especially pronounced compared to just a few minutes before (when, or immediately after eating), when you had so much energy from all the carbohydrates and sugar coursing through your body.

Revisiting my story briefly... During the workday, about 11:30 or 12, I'd have a rice-based lunch or a sandwich with large slices of bread. At about 2-3 pm, my energy level would drop significantly.

I'd start thinking about sweet tea or candy or some other carbohydrate-based snack. All these, I knew, would give me the perk I needed to be more alert and focused. Eventually, I'd find my way to the convenience store, where I'd get a sugar-fix. My taste buds were doing the happy dance and of course, that restored my energy for a while. But, I didn't realize how significant the consequences were.

Unfortunately those choices came with very regrettable consequences: a worse energy crash later, incessant sugar cravings, and an unusual plumpness to my belly and thighs: the dreaded weight gain.

Eating carbohydrates, even 'healthy' carbohydrates like whole-grains and brown rice, still means ingesting a form of sugar. Sugar, in all its forms, sets off the roller coaster of blood sugar and insulin, the resulting crash, and incorrigible sugar cravings.

It's no wonder consuming carbohydrates at lunch leads to a mid-afternoon slump, oftentimes accompanied by irritability or moodiness.

SODA

Coke, pop, soda, sweet tea, juice, and other forms of liquid sugar result in the same symptoms as eating too many carbohydrates: a rise in blood sugar, followed by a precipitous fall. These can be just as likely as edible carbohydrates or coffee to be causing your energy roller coaster throughout the day.

When you're sipping sugar-laden drinks slowly, thus ingesting your sugar over longer periods, you may indeed sustain high blood sugar. This allows you to temporarily avoid the 'crash.' But what goes up, must come down, including your energy. And if it doesn't, well, that's a recipe for metabolic syndrome, including diabetes. Once you're on a pre-diabetic path, you don't receive that same energy boost you used to because your muscles don't know how to use that sugar. The high just isn't the same. All around, drinking sugary drinks are going to lead to problems.

What about sugar-free "diet" soda?

Those 0-calorie, 0-carb, 0-sugar colas still contain upwards of 32-58 mg of caffeine per 20 ounces. While this caffeine level isn't as steep as a cup of coffee, you could still experience the same caffeine high and subsequent low as java drinkers.

Diet sodas are sweetened and preserved with aspartame, phosphoric acid, phenylalanine, and other additives with only questionable safety records. Some theorize that as your body, namely the liver, tries to interpret and then mobilize these chemical toxins out of circulation, it causes sluggishness and brain fog. This is because resources are being directed to the liver and kidneys to flush out the chemicals, directing blood and oxygen away from the brain, thus reducing productivity and mental focus.

Beyond that, research suggest that drinking diet soda, despite its calorie-free nature, leads to a faster expanding waistline, desensitized to fullness and sweet tastes, resulting in overeating and higher consumption sweet things, plus a higher risk of heart attack and stroke.[2] Here is another scary connection: aspartame has also been linked with dizziness, fatigue, migraines, and sleep disorders, which may precisely explain your mid-afternoon slump.

If you've checked your cup and checked your plate, and you're not filling up on caffeine or carbohydrates, yet you're still fatigued mid-afternoon, read on to find out other culprits.

Or, skip ahead to page nine for solutions to beating the 2 pm lull.

SLEEP

When you don't get enough quality sleep, you're bound to be more tired. Whether you have that heavy eyelid feeling throughout the day, or experience it more acutely mid-afternoon, that's a sign your body may be in need of more sleep.

With only moderate amount of sleep, most people can function 4-7 hours before they need more shut eye. That roughly corresponds with mid-afternoon.

Those who are severely sleep-deprived may not even make it through the morning. And any lack of quality sleep will affect performance, concentration, and memory.

If you're not getting 7-9 hours of quality shut eye, you're more likely to have a mid-afternoon crash.

NATURAL RHYTHM

The body has several natural rhythms that drive energy throughout the day. Many situations and factors in modern life can pull these rhythms out of order, leaving you feeling exhausted or the more worrisome, wired but tired feeling.

The most well-known of these is the circadian rhythm, which is largely governed by light exposure: rising sun in the morning means "time to wake up," while the darkness of evening signals "time to sleep." Circadian rhythm is very easily disrupted by viewing TV or computer screens at night or not being exposed to sunlight during the daytime, either of which can disrupt the sleep cycle.

Another key rhythm is governed by the hormone cortisol. In a healthy situation, cortisol is high in the morning, dropping mid-afternoon through evening to encourage sleep, and beginning to rise again in the middle of the night.

Cortisol also has an interplay with blood sugar. As we learned, insulin directs sugar out of the blood stream, storing it in muscles, fat, and the liver. Cortisol has the opposite effect on blood sugar: when the body needs more, it tells the liver and muscles to free up the sugar for immediate use. The primary cause of upended cortisol patterns is stress. Stress can come in many forms: physical, psychological/emotional, too much caffeine, intermittent fasting, deficiency of relaxing and rejuvenating practices, and much more.

Therefore, if you feel fatigued and out of energy all day, everyday (except for nighttime), your cortisol rhythm may be dysregulated, and you should get tested for adrenal complications.

In healthy individuals, cortisol levels begin to dip mid-afternoon as an early preparation for sleep. So, yes, it can be a good thing that your energy begins to slide a bit in the late afternoon--this reflects a healthy cortisol pattern.

Sociologically, the concept of a single sleep time, extending 7-9 hours, is a relatively new concept in human development.[3] Think of the siesta in Latin cultures, or looking even farther back in pre-electricity agricultural days, people would often have two sleeps to reflect the lack of available light.[4]

To some extent, natural biological rhythms encourage a mid-afternoon lull. In Part II, we'll look at ways to cope and minimize that impact, while improving productivity without compromising health.

Now that you have an understanding of what might be causing your mid-afternoon energy crash, let's see how we can minimize it, for better productivity, greater mental clarity, and stable energy, all without the negative effects of consuming sugary pick-me-ups or fancy late-in-the-day coffee drinks.

Part II

WHAT TO DO ABOUT YOUR AFTERNOON CRASH

DRINK TEA

Drinking tea, true tea from the *Camellia sinensis* plant, namely white, green, oolong, black or pu-erh, offers many of the benefits of coffee without the drawbacks. These teas are very popular in Asia, and have been for centuries, for this and many other reasons.

How?

Tea contains lower levels of caffeine plus the amino acid L-Theanine. While coffee or soda provides a quick jolt, followed by a steep decline due to its fast-acting caffeine, L-Theanine in tea offers a moderating effect. Let me explain.

An equal size cup of tea contains roughly ¼ to ½ the amount of caffeine in coffee, so in that regard, it's already less likely to send you into a tailspin of caffeine crash. Second, L-Theanine, an amino acid unique to tea, slows the release of caffeine, so the effect is more moderate.

Interestingly, research is connecting the combination of caffeine and L-Theanine with increased alpha wave activity in the brain, essentially improving clarity and inducing calmness, or simultaneous focus and relaxation.[5] Likewise, research suggests this pairing improves reaction time, memory, concentration, and ability to block out distractions.[6]

While there is a deficiency of research specifically testing the differences between two cups of coffee, 2 cups tea, or one of each in the morning, from the existing studies we can infer that even coffee addicts would do well to switch out at least one cup of coffee for tea. Besides less of a coffee crash, drinking tea means avoiding the jittery effects of coffee.

Because of its lower caffeine levels, plus the relaxation properties of L-Theanine, tea can also be drunk in the afternoon with fewer worries of sleepless nights. For that mid-afternoon time, tea will help you maintain energy, focus, and productivity.

SWITCH TO FAT AND PROTEIN-BASED MEALS

While fat has long been demonized by health organizations and mainstream media, it should be noted that fat is the only (significant) source of calories, nutrients, and sensations of fullness that doesn't affect blood sugar. carbohydrates cause a severe rise in blood sugar, and with (proper response to) insulin, an even quicker fall. Protein causes a slow, moderate rise in blood sugar, followed by an easy gentle decline. Fat has no such effect.

Therefore, to avoid a sugar crash, or even a 'complex-carbohydrate' crash after lunch (or any meal, for that matter), minimize consumption of carbohydrate-containing foods and drinks, and opt for protein and fat. When consuming meals of protein and fat, blood sugar and insulin will stay more stable, allowing for continuous, sustained energy. (Avoid overeating, especially if you have low stomach acid or depressed enzyme production, which can draw too much blood and resources away from the brain to use in digestion.)

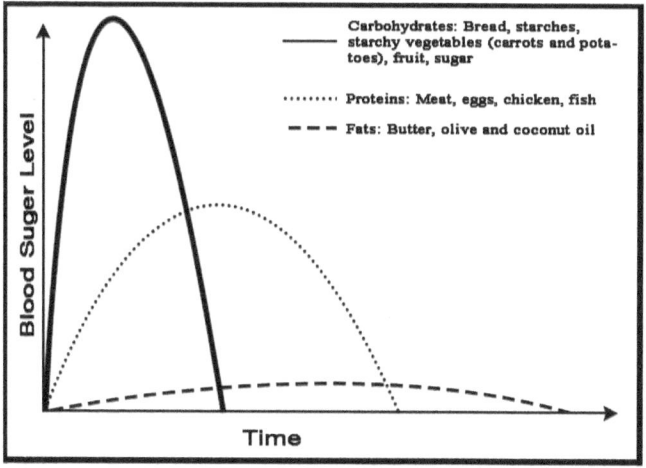

A brief word about choosing the right fats since eating fat is such a misunderstood and controversial topic. Wherever possible, opt for naturally-occurring fats, such as coconut oil, olives and olive oil, avocado, nuts, seeds, and fatty fish. Avoid transfats and other modern industrial fats like margarine, canola, soybean, and corn oil, as well as other vegetable oils, all of which are derived by chemical processing, are high in easily-oxidized polyunsaturated fats (PUFAs), and are pro-inflammatory.

Of course, skip the soda, punch, lemonade, sweet tea, or other primarily sugar drinks. The best choices to support stable blood sugar are water, unsweetened tea, or sparkling water, all of which can be flavored with lemon.

When blood sugar and insulin increase only modestly in response to eating, they support better energy balance for a longer period of time. This means afternoon energy is much more stable, focus is better, productivity can be higher, and alertness need not diminish.

To summarize, when you have an important meeting mid-afternoon that you need to be alert for, a critical project that must be finished, or a negotiation that requires your full cognitive abilities, stick with a light lunch composed primarily of leafy greens, protein, and fat. This will ensure digestion doesn't interfere with performance. Energy and focus will stay high, and satiety is maintained all afternoon.

SLEEP MORE OR TAKE A NAP

As we're constantly reminded in the media, sleep is very important to well-being, mental health, and a myriad of bodily functions. The same is true of sleep's impact on performance and alertness.

If you're hitting a wall mid-afternoon and it's not from the caffeine effect wearing off, the issue might be in getting enough quality sleep. The next time you're dozing off in a meeting, let this serve as a reminder to yourself to go to bed early, or find a way to take a power nap.

Increasing research is coming out demonstrating the benefits of brief naps on improving alertness, efficiency and productivity. In fact, many companies are starting to take note of these conclusions and are offering designated napping areas. If no such option exists in your workplace, consider going to your car for a cat nap, or closing your door and turning off your phone for a few minutes.

To learn how to optimize the benefits of your nap, whether that be for creative muscle, focus, or more energy, consult The Wall Street Journal[7] and lifehacker[8], which have both reported on the best ways to maximize efficiency and effectiveness of naps. Different times of the day, plus the length of the nap, can positively impact creativity, alertness, and cognitive memory. Balance these goals versus obligations and daily schedule.

Napping also feels more like embracing the natural rhythms of our body and our evolutionary history. It's also a lot better for body chemistry and composition (muscle v. fat), blood sugar control, and insulin management than reaching for a high-carbohydrate snack mid-afternoon.

Some world leaders and famous creative minds, including Winston Churchill, John F. Kennedy, and Salvador Dalí, are prime examples of people who slept midday to enhance cognitive performance and refresh their creativity.

Scientists also theorize that people who take quality naps, even when sleeping hours total less than 7, can perform just as well as people who sleep 8 hours nightly.

If napping isn't an option, work toward quieting your activities and the TV, dimming the lights, and getting to bed earlier, so you can get a full 8 hours of sleep in anticipation of an alert, productive next day.

MOVE YOUR BODY AND GO OUTSIDE

When sitting for a long time, you feel more likely to doze off than if you were standing or walking, right? This is because the body has sunk into conservation mode and doesn't need to work as hard to circulate blood. Sometimes this goes too far, marginally depriving key organs of oxygen, hence the yawn. Low levels of oxygen in the body, and especially the brain, make us feel lethargic and sleepy.

To combat this, move your body. Increase blood flow by going for a walk and swinging your arms. Do a few pushups, squats, or bicep curls. You'll get the blood moving, increasing oxygen flow to the whole body, and it's a quick stimulant-free way to wake up. Why do you think morning exercise is so popular?

Better yet, take your walk outside. Walking outside during the daytime has the added benefit of increasing exposure to the sun, which helps with circadian rhythm calibration, reduces Seasonal Affective Disorder, and provides a source of Vitamin D, a powerful immunoregulatory agent.

The Japanese also believe that walking outside, near plants in nature, offers the additional benefit of exposure to ions in the air that restore energy, enhance cognitive ability, and increase stamina. The understanding is that indoor air becomes devoid of these ions, which causes drowsiness, lost productivity, and poor focus, hence why office workers often feel blah. The Japanese remedy this situation, and as a result, work some of the longest days of any nation, by putting machines in every office that replenish the ions in the air.

But you don't need to worry about the technology, just go outside for a few minutes of brisk walking, deep breathing, and perhaps throw in a few lunges, pushups, or stretches. Even Ralph Waldo Emerson and Henry David Thoreau, over 100 years ago, knew the value of nature to the creative brain. Stop and smell the flowers.

By the time you come back inside, you'll be more alert, your head will be clear, and you'll again be ready to focus.

My Solution

To wrap up my story... For a long time, before I had the understanding and knowledge I've shared with you in this book, I struggled! After months, even 2-3 years, of carbohydrate-heavy lunches, followed by mid-afternoon crashes, curtailed only by sugary afternoon pick-me-ups, and the frustrating, incessant carbohydrate cravings and weight gain, I decided enough was enough!

I sought help. I went to my Chinese Medicine doctor, lamenting my sorry state and seeking a solution.

What I thought would be an easy, quick-fix turned into nearly two years of studying Chinese medicine, working with expert Traditional Chinese Medicine herbalists to develop and produce the 'easy' solution I envisioned from the beginning.

Commencing this studying, I discovered that almost never are there easy answers to health questions. As I wrapped up my studies in Hangzhou, China, I went on to India and Bali, Indonesia, embarking on a journey delving into the traditional healing practices of these regions.

In India, I explored the wisdom of the ancient yogis, known as Ayurveda, including lifestyle practices that vary according to the season and time of day, as well as herbs and massage.

Bali, too makes use of medicinal plants, but places a greater emphasis on energy healing, and the use of intention and the power of belief, to achieve a desired outcome, thus incorporating a spiritual aspect to all healing.

As I concluded my overseas studies, my original frustration with low afternoon energy still weighed on my mind and I continued to envision a simpler answer. By wrapping together all that I'd learned over the years, I created the packaged solution I sought in the beginning, and I named it Belight Tea.

Belight Tea is ideal for those long days at the office, especially for those who don't necessarily have the wherewithal to immediately make lifestyle changes. You can read more about what makes Belight Tea particularly effective for the mid-afternoon slump on our website.[9]

While I'm very proud of Belight Tea and the positive feedback it's received from people all around the world, my studies taught me the value and advantages of lifestyle changes. That's why I've written this guide for you: to provide a broad, well-rounded understanding of the afternoon slump and the actions you can take to minimize it in your own life.

Part III

MAKING IT WORK FOR YOU

Here's what you can do next to apply what you learned in this guide to making those afternoons not feel like so much of a slump:

- If you're a morning coffee drinker, begin by replacing 1 cup of coffee with a cup of tea. (Note: Herbal teas are caffeine-free.)

- Ditch the soda, juice, and other sweet drinks. Water, sparkling water, or unsweetened tea will serve you much better.

- Take note of your lunch. If the largest item is a starch, grain, or other fast-acting carbohydrate with no fiber, consider eliminating that to favor fat and protein. If going starch-free isn't possible, try cutting it in half: only have one slice of bread on the sandwich, half the amount of pasta or rice, or skip the bread that comes with your salad. Note: Salad is a good choice, but some dressings are loaded with sugar (and will cause the same blood sugar spike), so ask for it on the side or go with vinegar and olive oil.

- Add more healthy fats to your lunch to slow blood sugar and insulin rise. Good choices are olive oil, coconut oil, avocado oil, nuts and seeds, avocado, and fish.

- Cinnamon is also thought to moderate the blood sugar/insulin effects of carbohydrates. This is a nice addition to tea or full-fat Greek yogurt and can be used liberally.

- Count how many hours you sleep in a 24 hour period. If it's significantly less than 8 hours, consider ways you can get more sleep, even if that's a 15-minute power nap in your car at lunch time, or perhaps before dinner.

- Continue to repeat and refine the above steps.

- Consider drinking Belight Tea as you make the transition to a more alert, focused, productive you with stable energy and good concentration throughout the day.

- Of course, you can always take a walk outside, notice the fragrances of nature, swing your arms, breathe deep and let the oxygen flow in to revitalize you. This is also a great way to have a productive meeting: walking and fresh air stimulate creative thinking.

- For days when the sleep angel or troll of lethargy just keeps overtaking you, and napping isn't an option, it's good to have Belight Tea handy. It'll help you avoid the sugar trap, keep you going, and encourage balance.

CHECKLIST TO PREVENTING THE AFTERNOON SLUMP

DO:

☐ Switch to tea after 1 cup of coffee

☐ Drink only water or unsweetened tea

☐ Reduce sugar, starches, and grains

☐ Try to keep total carbohydrates under 30g per meal, and make sure at least half of that is fiber

☐ Be cautious of hidden sugars, such as those in salad dressing

☐ Choose healthy fats such as coconut oil, olive oil, avocado, or fish

☐ Have protein and healthy fats with every meal to slow insulin response

☐ Get at least 7-8 hours of sleep per night

☐ Allow yourself the luxury of a nap if you haven't slept enough

☐ Add cinnamon to tea, yogurt, etc

☐ Visit BelightTea.com to stock up on Belight for tough afternoons

☐ Exercise lightly with simple moves or light stretching

☐ Take a walk outside

☐ Get close to nature and breathe deeply

DON'T:

- ☐ Keep pounding the coffee to 'fuel you through'
- ☐ Drink soda or diet soda
- ☐ Get sugary drinks like lemonade, punch, or sweet tea
- ☐ Believe an energy drink is better
- ☐ Eat a pasta dish, pizza, or bread-heavy sandwich at lunch
- ☐ Overeat at lunch, which can also make you groggy
- ☐ Snack on donuts, cookies, or other sugar-filled junk
- ☐ Let the vending machine be your only food source-- it's just junk!
- ☐ Consume bad fats
- ☐ Be afraid to include healthy fats with every meal
- ☐ Skimp on protein or high-fiber vegetables
- ☐ Shortchange your sleep
- ☐ Believe you're different and can thrive on only 5 hours of sleep
- ☐ Feel guilty taking a nap if circumstances dictate it
- ☐ Ignore the benefits of tea, including L-theanine

A FINAL WORD

As you're now at the end of this book, if you liked it and found it helpful, I encourage you to share the book with others. Feel free to give or lend them this copy.

Or, if you prefer, please post the link below on Facebook, Twitter, Pinterest, Reddit, or whatever social platform you use. Even if your version of social is email, pass along the link to others who'd be interested.

http://bit.ly/Mid-Afternoon

My goal is to support people like you to be their most productive, alert, and aware, to have energy and mental clarity so they can be successful in following their dreams and supporting their family. This helps you and everyone live the best possible life.

With your share, I can reach more people. Thank you.

If you have any questions or feedback about this guide, you can email me at Toffler@WorldVitae.com.

REFERENCES

1. "Caffeine Metabolism." *Caffeine Informer.* http://www.caffeineinformer.com/caffeine-metablolism

2. Firestone, Tasha. "Drinking Diet Soda is Dangerous to Your Health." *Freak of Nature Fitness.* http://www.freakofnaturefitness.com/blog/2012/08/27/Stop-Drinking-Diet-Soda.aspx

3. Hegarty, Stephanie. "The myth of the eight-hour sleep." *BBC News Magazine.* http://www.bbc.co.uk/news/magazine-16964783

4. Barton, Laura. "Sleep: why they used to do it twice a night." *The Guardian.* http://www.theguardian.com/commentisfree/2012/feb/24/sleep-twice-a-night-anxiety

5. Nobre AC; Rao A; Owen GN. "L-theanine, a

natural constituent in tea, and its effect on mental state." *Asia Pacific Journal of Clinical Nutrition.* 2008; 17 Suppl 1:167-8. http://www.ncbi.nlm.nih.gov/pubmed/18296328

6. Haskell CF; Kennedy DO; Milne AL; Wesnes KA; Scholey AB. "The effects of L-theanine, caffeine and their combination on cognition and mood." *Biology Psychology.* 2008 Feb;77(2):113-22. Epub 2007 Sep 26. http://www.ncbi.nlm.nih.gov/pubmed/18006208

7. Reddy, Sumathi. "The Perfect Nap: Sleeping Is a Mix of Art and Science." *The Wall Street Journal.*
    http://online.wsj.com/news/articles/SB10001424127887323932604579050990895301888

8. Pinola, Melanie. "Calculate the Best Time to Nap with this Interactive Nap Wheel." *lifehacker.*
    http://lifehacker.com/5874738/calculate-the-best-time-to-nap-with-this-interactive-nap-wheel

9. Niemuth, Toffler. "How Belight Tea Eases the Afternoon Slump." *Belight Tea.*
    http://belighttea.com/belight-tea-eases-afternoon-slump/

ABOUT THE AUTHOR

In her first published book, wellness educator, speaker, and entrepreneur, Toffler Niemuth, draws on her own experience as well as that of countless others who lament the same problem. The result is this book, written after many years of learning about and trying to understand the complex factors that result in low energy mid-afternoon.

Exploring nutrition and fitness for over 15 years, and later yoga, fasting, health and wellness, Toffler is passionate about discovering solutions and helping people improve their health in the unique way that makes sense for them. She has a B.S. from the University of Southern California, certificates from Zhejiang Chinese Medicine University, Greens Ayur Center, is a trained yoga teacher, and herbalist. Toffler fell in love with tea during her six years living in Asia, five of which were in Mainland China, sipping her way through all styles of tea and tisanes.

Drawing on her love of tea, fascination with herbs, and trying to solve the issues connected with her afternoon slump, Toffler developed Belight Tea. Belight Tea is sophisticated blend of pu-erh tea and five Chinese medicine herbs that support energy to minimize the afternoon lull, soothe digestion, reduce stress, cravings, and snacking, and aid weight control. More information about Toffler and Belight Tea can be found on the website: http://BelightTea.com

www.ingramcontent.com/pod-product-compliance
Lightning Source LLC
Chambersburg PA
CBHW021210290526
45796CB00005B/30